RICE DIET FOR HEALTHY LIFESTYLE

Transform Your Health with Delicious Rice-Based Recipes and Lifestyle Tips

Kayson J. Liam

1

TABLE OF CONTENTS

CHAPTER ONE

INTRODUCTION

The rice diet is a low-fat, low-protein, high-carbohydrate weight-loss plan. The diet, which emphasizes mindfulness, lower sodium intake, and calorie deficit, may assist some people in improving their health and losing weight.

Walter Kempner, a 1934 graduate of Duke University's Department of Medicine and a 1903 German native, is credited with creating the rice diet.

Kempner looked into how diet affected conditions like diabetes and hypertension and discovered that those who consumed rice as a primary food rarely had issues with these conditions.

Kempner created a rice, fruit, juice, sugar, and vitamin and iron supplement diet to assist treat these and other linked health issues.

According to Kempner's theory, changing a person's food and way of life could save their lives by lowering the amount of work their kidneys had to do.

Since 1939, more than 18,000 people from all over the world who suffer from diabetes, obesity, heart disease, and hypertension have been treated with the Kempner diet, often known as the rice diet, frequently with remarkable results.

Rice is a staple food for about 3.5 billion people globally, most of whom live in Asia, Latin America, and certain parts of Africa. The majority of individuals follow some form of rice diet. For example, in South Asia, rice is a staple food. Similar to this, sushi—tiny pieces of raw fish wrapped in rice—is served with every meal in Japan.

Rice is a staple component in a plethora of well-liked, delectable recipes. Therefore, it wouldn't be incorrect to argue that rice is the most widely consumed food in the world.

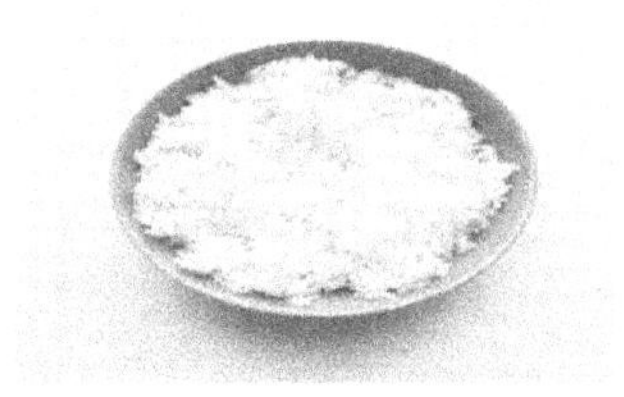

However, is rice rich in nutrients? And is losing weight possible with a rice diet plan? Continue reading to find out the responses to each of these questions and more.

CHAPTER TWO

TYPES OF RICE

Rice is divided into four categories by these four main factors:

Kernel dimensions

Tastes

Level of milling, and

Starch composition

These variables have led experts to identify over 12,000 different types of rice. The most well-liked and often utilized of these are as follows:

Rice with Arborio

Rice Sushi

Basmati Rice

Grain Brown Rice

Blanched Rice

Forgotten Rice

The Jasmine Rice

Rice with Black Color

The Best Type of Rice to Help You Lose Weight

The greatest rice to consume when attempting to reduce weight is brown rice. They are a low-carb diet that are lower in calories and provide vital nutrients, making them the perfect substitute for white rice while trying to lose weight.

Unprocessed rice is generally recommended for diets aimed at weight loss. Red rice, black rice, brown rice, and wild rice are the options available to you.

Grain size is also a significant factor. Because long grain is less starchy and less sweet than short and medium grain, it is better for weight loss.

Effectiveness of Rice Food for Losing Weight

You won't be able to lose weight on rice alone. Still, it ought to be a component of any well-rounded program for losing weight.

Research indicates that rice can be a beneficial addition to a diet, despite the fact that simple carbohydrates have historically been avoided in weight control programs. You have to be extremely strict about the kind, quantity, cooking method, and additions of rice if you want it to be an efficient diet for weight loss.

To help you lose weight, try these suggestions for cooking and consuming brown rice:

•	Instead of fried rice, use steamed or boiled rice.

•	Before cooking, soak and wash well three or four times.

•	Rice should be combined with high-fiber vegetables to make a balanced meal that promotes weight loss.

•	You may cook brown rice with coconut water rather than just regular water to make it taste better.

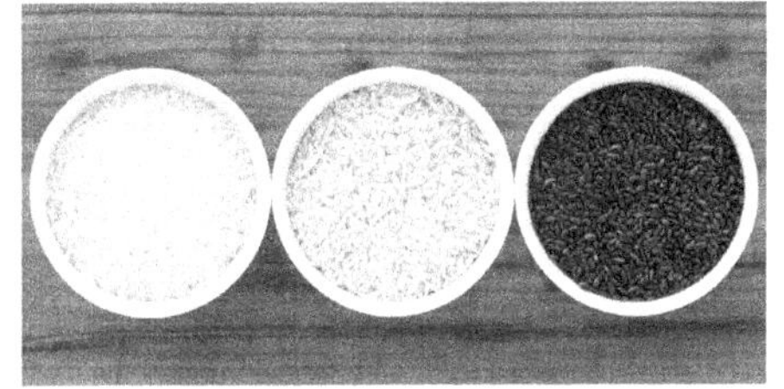

CHAPTER THREE

ADVANTAGES OF A RICE DIET THAT MAY EXIST

Males can lose an average of 30 pounds in the first four weeks of the diet, while females can lose an average of 19 pounds. The diet is said to help people lose weight swiftly and safely.

They also assert that a rice diet increases vitality and mental clarity.

The following factors make the diet successful in promoting weight loss:

- Because salt stimulates the appetite, cutting back on it can lead to weight loss from both water retention and overindulgence.

- The diet reduces saturated fats and increases fiber-rich carbs to help keep people feeling full.

- Because the diet consists primarily of low-calorie foods, cutting calories is easier.

There are four more crucial strategies to ensure the diet is successful.

- Eating with awareness and knowing what nutrients are in the food.

- Letting down and scheduling time for exercises like tai chi, journaling, or mindful breathing.

- Doing frequent physical activity.

- Locating relationships and networks of support.

HERE ARE SOME MORE FANTASTIC HEALTH BENEFITS OF EATING RICE

•   Brown rice offers long-term disease prevention.

Due to its ability to maintain the bran layer, brown rice has defensive substances known as flavonoids, such as quercetin and apigenin. These substances are vital in the fight against illness. Wholegrains, such as brown rice, have been associated in numerous studies to a lower risk of heart disease, type 2 diabetes, and some malignancies, including stomach and pancreatic tumors.

•   After physical activity, white rice replenishes glycogen stores and boosts energy.

White rice is frequently the favored energy source for athletes, particularly when they are refueling after a workout. This is true because white rice and other refined carbohydrates provide an easy-to-access, fast-acting source of the carbohydrate needed to restore muscle glycogen following physical activity.

•	Natural Anti-Inflammatory and Gluten-Free: Do you have sensitivity to gluten? Not only is rice delicious, but it is also free of gluten!

It may surprise you to learn that rice is the most widely consumed grain free of gluten. This is particularly valid for those with celiac disease. It functions as our bodies' natural anti-inflammatory, which is always rather advantageous.

You can safely include rice in your diet even if you have gluten sensitivity. Your digestive system won't become inflamed because it is gluten-free. Rice is a fantastic addition to any diet because it's crucial to continually look for strategies to minimize inflammation throughout our bodies.

- Encourages Heart Health

Have you been trying to think of natural ways to strengthen your heart? If so, a regular rice diet can be the solution you've been searching for!

Rice naturally reduces inflammation, as was previously established. Because of its anti-inflammatory qualities, it helps to slow down the rate at which atherosclerotic plaque deposits inside blood vessel walls. Consequently, this lowers your chance of developing serious cardiac issues including heart attacks or strokes.

While brown rice and white rice offer similar advantages, brown rice is superior. This is because brown rice has the husk, which is where the majority of the nutrients are found. Another excellent resource for enhancing heart health is rice bran oil.

Because of its many antioxidant qualities, rice bran oil lowers cholesterol levels in the body and eventually improves cardiovascular health.

• Has the potential to lower the risk of cancer development

Do you want to continue taking preventative measures against the risk of cancer? Eating rice and other high-fiber meals lowers your risk of developing cancer!

The high fiber content of rice facilitates better digestion and lowers blood pressure. You receive better overall physical wellness in exchange. Also, maintaining a healthy digestive system prevents the body's waste from being stagnant for extended periods of time.

Maintaining the flow reduces the possibility that this waste may come into contact with the body's healthy cells. This is beneficial in the prevention and treatment of colorectal and intestinal cancers. However, rice's fight against cancer doesn't end there.

- Controls blood sugar & blood pressure

Do you experience elevated blood pressure? Are you trying to find natural solutions to lower your blood pressure? If so, you might want to think about include rice in your diet!

Managing Blood Pressure

Eating rice can help those with hypertension manage their condition. It has relatively little sodium in it. It is well known that sodium causes the body's veins and arteries to narrow.

When you do this, your blood pressure rises and the cardiovascular system is under more stress or strain. Sodium has long-term effects on the heart and can lead to a number of heart problems. Maintaining a low-sodium diet lowers these risks.

Managing Blood Sugar

However, rice also has a hypoglycemic effect. While both brown and white rice can control blood sugar levels, brown rice is a better option for this advantage. Brown rice is superior in slowing down the body's absorption of glucose because it has more fiber in the husk.

The body's insulin has more time to correctly distribute the glucose throughout the body since the body absorbs glucose more slowly.

Potential dangers

The rice diet may be difficult or too restrictive for certain people, which could lead to problems while dining out and potential nutritional deficiencies.

For instance, a low protein diet may prevent certain persons from gaining muscle mass or from having the amino acids needed to synthesis protein. Furthermore, limiting good fats could have negative health effects because the body requires them for proper operation.

I will advise anyone taking medication for high blood pressure, diabetes, or congestive heart failure to speak with their doctor before starting the diet.

The dosage of certain drugs, such as warfarin and lithium, may need to be changed by a doctor. The diet should also not be followed by those who have undergone ureteral diversion surgeries, colon surgery, or decreased kidney function.

If someone is on the rice diet and has lightheadedness or nausea, they should consult a physician. For vegans and vegetarians, the rice diet works well, however it may require the use of supplements for

omega-3 fatty acids and vitamin
B12.

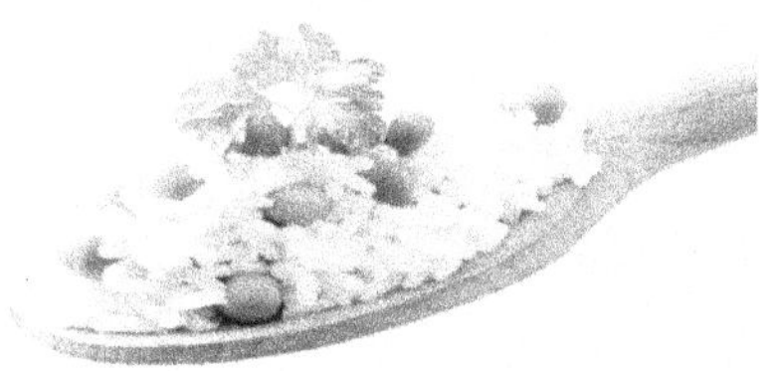

23

CHAPTER FOUR

MENU FOR THE RICE DIET

Three diet phases—detox, weight loss, and maintenance of the weight loss—are explained here. The diet calls for increasing daily caloric intake by a small amount, from around 1,000 to over 1,200. The meal plans provide serving sizes, so there's no need to keep track of calories, the authors point out.

A person's daily calorie intake should consist of 1,000–1200 calories, plus any fruits or vegetables they choose to consume. However, they shouldn't enhance their meals with more fat.

It is advised by the diet that individuals take in 500–1000 mg of salt day, with a daily minimum of

300 mg. For those who don't eat dairy, two slices of ordinary bread or an additional 200 mg of salt from another source should be consumed to ensure appropriate intake.

See your doctor if you're worried about how much sodium you're consuming. After that, they can adhere to the rice diet as closely as they feel comfortable or able to while still trying to maintain their salt intake within the parameters that they and their healthcare provider have agreed upon.

The diet advises following certain serving sizes from various dietary groups, such as vegetables, protein, and carbohydrates. Rice, beans, and cereal are examples of carbohydrates. A perfect example of animal products are fish and poultry. Vegetarian items include beans and eggs.

The following portion amounts are recommended by the diet:

•   Just one starch A quarter to a cup of cereal (not low sodium), one slice of bread, half a cup of cooked pasta or other grains, or one-third cup of cooked rice or beans

•   One dairy product without fat: One cup of nonfat soy, yogurt, fortified grain milk, or cow's milk

•   One vegetable, or one cup of uncooked veggies

•   One fruit: one cup of grapes, one medium-sized fruit, or one cup of chopped fruit

•   One condiment is one teaspoon (tsp) honey or maple

syrup. Herbs and salt spices are prohibited in the diet.

Any fruit, grain, or vegetable may be consumed by dieters as long as no additional fat or salt is added. You may have one teaspoon of honey or maple syrup per day.

The three phases are guided by the following:

PHASE 1: DETOX

This stage entails ridding the body of extra water weight, toxins, and sodium. For a week, people should adhere to phase one.

The following are part of the phase one diet:

Adopt a simple rice diet for one day a week. This consists of two fruits and two starches for breakfast, lunch, and dinner.

Six days a week, eat rice that is lacto-vegetarian.

- One carbohydrate, one nonfat dairy, and one fruit for breakfast

- Three grains, three veggies, and one fruit for lunch

- Three carbohydrates, three veggies, and one fruit for dinner

For six days a week, here's an example of breakfast:

- One-quarter to one cup of cereal made from whole grains.

- One cup Greek yogurt without fat

- Three scallions

PHASE 2: WEIGHT LOSS

This stage seeks to assist an individual in reaching their specific weight loss objectives. The amount of weight that someone wishes to reduce will determine how long phase two lasts. According to the authors, combining this phase with consistent exercise can help someone lose 3.5 pounds (lbs) each week or 14 pounds per month on average.

Every weekday, follow this simple rice diet consisting of two starches and two vegetables for breakfast, lunch, and dinner.

Five days a week, rice diet high in lacto-vegetablesy

•   One carbohydrate, one nonfat dairy, and one fruit for breakfast

- Three grains, three veggies, and one fruit for lunch

- Three carbohydrates, three veggies, and one fruit for dinner

For one day a week. The vegetarian plus rice diet, which has 200 extra calories and includes protein compared to the lacto-vegetarian rice diet.

- Two carbohydrates and one fruit for breakfast

- Lunch consists of three grains, three veggies, and one fruit.

- Supper consists of three carbohydrates, three proteins (or two dairy products), three vegetables, and one fruit.

Five days a week, here's an example of lunch:

- One cup of cooked rice or beans, or one and a half cups of any other cooked pasta or grain

- Tomato sauce, half a cup

- Mandarin orange and spinach salad (2.5 cups) with 2 tablespoons balsamic dressing

PHASE 3: MAINTENANCE

This stage aids in the maintenance of the new weight. A person may choose to add 200 calories to their diet after reaching their goal weight, which could include dairy products, seafood, or healthy fats like nuts and avocados.

- One day per week, follow a simple rice diet consisting of two starches and two fruits for breakfast, lunch, and dinner.

Four days a week: rice diet high in lacto-vegetables

- One fruit, one carbohydrate, and one nonfat dairy for breakfast

- Lunch is three grains, three veggies, and one fruit.

- Dinner is three grains, three veggies, and one fruit.

Two days a week: rice-plus-vegetarian diet

- Two starches and one fruit for breakfast

- Lunch is three grains, three veggies, and one fruit.

- Supper consists of 3 carbohydrates, 3 proteins (or 2 dairy products), 3 veggies, and 1 fruit.

For two days a week, an example of a vegetarian meal with rice might be:

- Crispy flounder

- One cup of red potatoes with garlic and peel

- One-quarter cup of corn from the Southwest

- Salad in a cup with balsamic dressing

- One cup of spinach, creamed

- One orange or two clementines.

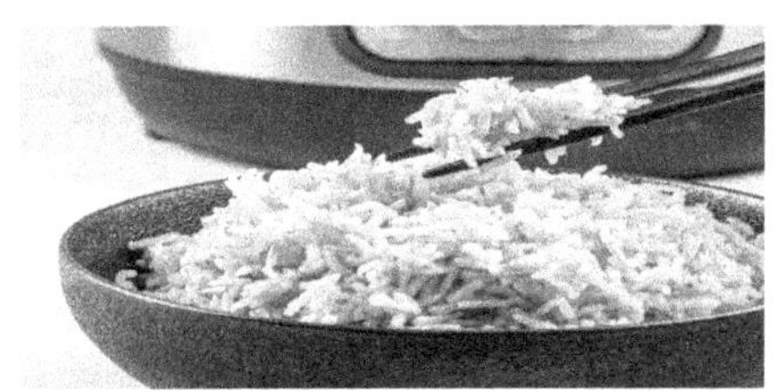

CHAPTER FIVE

WHAT WOULD A 7-DAY RICE DIET PLAN INCLUDE?

When following a diet plan, you need to pay close attention to how much food you eat at each meal. It would also be beneficial if you deliberately worked to burn off more calories than you take in. Doing physical activities such as swimming, running, or other sports is a great method to do this.

You are not need to restrict your 7-day rice diet plan to only rice. Rice should be a part of your diet, but only in moderation. Eat brown rice instead of white rice. Furthermore, deciding on the kind of diet you need to follow depends largely on your BMI score.

Your healthy weight is determined by your body mass index, or BMI, which takes into account your height. It tells you how likely it is that you will have health problems due to your weight. It also provides you with a clear understanding of your daily energy needs, your optimal body weight, and the healthy range of weights.

•	Whole grains: If you need carbohydrates, primarily brown rice

•	Fruits and vegetables: To meet your needs for fiber

•	Nuts and seeds: Provides good fats

- Again, healthy fats: homemade desi ghee and seed oils (olive, mustard, etc.).

- For the required amount of protein, use lentils, legumes, paneer, soy, tofu, etc.

It is usually advisable to speak with your nutritionist and doctor for a more comprehensive strategy.

Which Kind of Rice Helps You Lose Weight?

When trying to reduce weight, brown rice is the healthiest type of rice to eat! Due to their low calorie content and provision of essential nutrients, they are the perfect substitute for white rice when it comes to weight loss.

What is the ideal daily amount of rice to eat?

Each person may require a different amount of calories to lose weight, depending on a number of factors such as gender, build, height, and level of activity.

For women seeking to lose weight, a serving should typically contain about 37 grams of rice, and for males, it should contain about 50 grams.

Is rice suitable for all?

While reports have connected rice to elevated levels of arsenic contamination—which, over time, has been associated with a higher risk of cancer and heart disease— rice is still a basic food. Because the bran of the grain is where arsenic tends to accumulate the most, wholegrain rice may have more of this heavy metal pollutant than white rice.

Children are especially vulnerable to arsenic exposure because of their lesser body weight. Their restricted diet options and the fact that a lot of first foods are made with rice raise this danger. For this reason, all children under the age of five should not consume rice milk, which is formed from the grain's bran.

Some helpful cooking advice, like cleaning rice before using it and heating it with a lot of water, can help lower arsenic levels. Having said that, most people shouldn't have any issues with rice when it's consumed in moderation as part of a varied and balanced diet.

Please get advice from a licensed dietician or your general practitioner if you are worried.

Things on the rice diet list to eat

The rice diet has a lot of limitations. During this diet, you'll be eating:

Recent fruit

Produce

Minimal-salt beans

Whole grains

Slim-down protein

Dairy products without fat

To Keep Away

Junk food

Pop

Fruits in bottles

Cans

Milk chocolate.

Refrigerated food

Deep-fried cuisine

Prepared meals

Foods high in trans fats, processed sugar, and refined flour

You will have to give up junk food and make healthier dietary and lifestyle decisions.

What More Can You Do To Boost Your Health?

• You need to look after your sleeping schedule. One of the reasons for the accumulation of toxins in the body is sleep deprivation. Your DNA is altered by the dangerous free oxygen radicals, which can lead to a number of health issues like diabetes, heart disease, and obesity.

• Every day, spend at least five minutes in meditation. As you get more comfortable, extend the duration.

• Stay away from alcohol. 30 milliliters of wine are permitted once every week.

• Engage in regular exercise. From the first day of exercise, you will notice an improvement in your energy and mood.

- Make sure, you consume two or more liters of water. To improve the taste of your water bottle, you can add cucumber, ginger, mint leaves, and citrus fruits.

- Eat in consistent intervals. You will only deteriorate mentally, physically, and cognitively if you embark on a hunger strike.

It is evident that maintaining a healthy lifestyle in addition to a diet is necessary to stay in shape and be happy. You could, however, stick to a less stringent diet for that.

Who Is Appropriate For The Rice Diet?

This diet is appropriate for you to follow if:

You have hypertension.

Diabetes affects you.

You have cardiac problems.

Chronic renal failure is what you have.

You have elevated cholesterol.

You have a gluten sensitivity. It is true that rice has a low potassium content, making it the perfect food for people with higher potassium levels in their bodies.

Note:

You should ONLY adhere to this diet if your physician gives the all-clear.

CHAPTER SIX

FAQs

- Can eating rice help you lose weight?

In around ten weeks, males can lose roughly thirty pounds and women can lose twenty pounds by eating rice in moderation, exercising, and restricting their calorie intake. Individual differences exist in weight loss, though.

- Is eating rice a daily meal acceptable?

In moderation, eating rice on a daily basis is OK. Overindulgence in it could raise your risk of cardiovascular disease and type 2 diabetes.

- Are rice and eggs a healthy combination?

Yes, rice and eggs are good for you. They have the ideal ratio of protein to carbs. Consume in moderation, nevertheless, to prevent any unfavorable side effects, such as weight gain.

- Pasta versus rice: which is healthier?

Pasta made from whole wheat is a better option than rice. Instead of refined pasta, though, try rice.

- Does rice reduce inflammation?

Rice varieties like brown and wild have anti-inflammatory qualities. Their high fiber content helps to lessen inflammation. White rice might not aid in reducing inflammation, though, as it lacks fiber.

•   Is rice a more healthful food than bread?

Bread lacks some minerals and vitamins, which are found in rice, particularly brown rice. But whole grain bread is a better option if you're trying to cut back on calories and carbs.

•   Are diets based only on rice and beans healthy?

Because it is high in fiber, protein, and other vital vitamins and nutrients, a diet plan consisting solely of rice and beans is indeed healthful. A study found that eating rice with black, pinto, or dark red kidney beans may help persons with type 2 diabetes have a lower glycemic response.

TAKEAWAY

The fundamental calorie deficit, low fat content, and whole food nature of the rice diet may help some people lose weight effectively. When combined with regular exercise and lifestyle strategies like journaling, mindfulness, and community support, the rice diet may help people make lifestyle changes and live a healthier and more focused life.

People should prepare a more balanced meal during the maintenance phase and be mindful that following the rice diet exclusively for an extended period of time may result in nutrient shortages. Furthermore, because everyone has a different metabolism and state of health, what works for one person could not work for another.

You must be well-versed in the effects of the rice diet on weight loss and general health by this point. Please do not hesitate to contact a health professional if you would want further information.

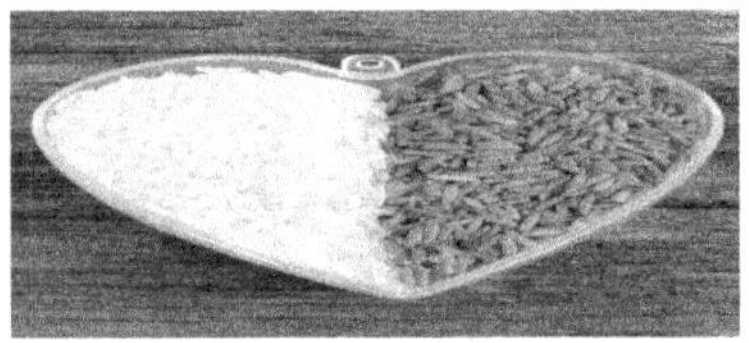

THE END

49

www.ingramcontent.com/pod-product-compliance
Lightning Source LLC
Chambersburg PA
CBHW051711250726
48653CB00007B/2975